Negotiating the process of having an Alzheimer's Dementia diagnosis in the family is often confusing and frustrating. This book connects with the experience of the loved ones of an individual with Alzheimer's Dementia, and it is an empathic and helpful guide in understanding and negotiating the process of recognizing, diagnosing, treating, and coping with a loved one with Alzheimer's Dementia.

Dr. Robert G. Arias, PhD
Arias Neuropsychology & Behavioral Medicine, PC

An Alzheimer or dementia diagnosis for you or your loved one poses a lot of unknowns. As a director of a memory care community, I know firsthand how difficult it can be for families to navigate. There are multiple paths this disease takes, and no one person's journey is the same. Learning as much as you can about the disease helps you solve everyday issues and improve quality of life for both you and your loved one. This book is an excellent and practical guide to help you navigate this tough challenge from the beginning to the end, providing practical advice, scenarios, support, and additional resources for you and your family.

Suzy Nootz, MSN, RN, CDP
Country House Residence for Memory Care

I Love Someone with Dementia ... So Why Am I Losing My Mind?

A Practical Guide

Beth Friesen
RN, CCM, CSA, CDP, CADDCT

INFUSIONMEDIA
Lincoln, Nebraska

Infusionmedia

2124 Y St, Flat #138

Lincoln, NE 68503

https://infusion.media

Printed in the United States

10 9 8 7 6 5 4 3 2 1

First Edition

Print ISBN: 978-1-945834-08-0

Ebook ISBN: 978-1-945834-10-3

Library of Congress Control Number: 2019910045

*This book is dedicated to the woman who taught me
everything, except how to live without her.
I love you, Mom, and pray I can be even half of what you
were to everyone who knew you.*

Ellen Margaret Thimm Esau
1929–2014

Contents

Preface

How did it begin for you? In our family, we went through theories to explain it all away...

"Well, she is in her late seventies."
"Maybe it's hormones."
"Could her carotid arteries be blocked?"
"Is she having blood pressure problems?"

Back and forth we went between thinking something was wrong and then talking to her a day later and concluding that, indeed, there was nothing wrong at all. It must certainly all be in our imagination. This game went on for at least a year or two before one day, while standing in line to pick up a pizza to feed my young family, it clicked.

Mom had Alzheimer's.

My three sisters and I were quickly on the same page. After all, three of us were nurses, and the other worked with a geriatric population on a daily basis. However, our dad was only not on the same page, he wasn't even reading the same book. Denial is a powerful force in dealing with dementia, and our dad had a strong case of it. At least another eighteen months passed before we finally convinced him that she needed to be evaluated.

Unfortunately, when she was diagnosed with "dementia, likely Alzheimer's" in March 2010, she was already well into the moderate stages of the disease. The opportunities to have conversations with her about her disease and what she would want in terms of care and end-of-life wishes was lost. The finality of the diagnosis was overwhelming and staggering, even for us as daughters who "knew" years before. And for our dad, it was catastrophic.

As daughters, we had a need to learn more about this disease and how we could best help Mom and be a support to our dad. I called a nonprofit group that was recommended by her physicians. From them, we basically got a list of support groups, the website address (for the nonprofit itself), and then were wished the best of luck. One of my sisters and dad attended a support group at one point and found it to be a gripe session for people to vent about being a caregiver. We found that to be no help whatsoever.

Later, my dad and I attended what was supposed to be an educational meeting at a local nonmedical in-home-care provider's office. They went through the definitions, diagnosis, stages, and pharmaceutical interventions that were currently offered. My dad only found that to be depressing and overwhelming. No real information was gathered there, either. We desperately wanted to know **how** best to take care of her and **how** best to support our dad, her primary caregiver.

This book is meant to be a guide to help you and those you love navigate this overwhelming diagnosis, and the months and years that follow. It includes what we wish we had known, what we learned, and the resources that helped us along the way. Included are also the discussions we all need to have, since none of us are getting out of this human experience alive. It is very important that you understand that there is no possible way I can cover every possible scenario in this book. What you do need to know, however, is that you can find the resources and people to help you.

1

Dementia and Alzheimer's Basics

VINCE LOMBARDI IS probably the most famous football coach in history. The Super Bowl trophy is named in his honor. But every year at the beginning of the season, he would approach his team the same way. He would hold up a football and proclaim, "Gentlemen, this is a football." He started at the beginning and with the basics. In order to start us off on the right foot, I believe we need to do the same. We all need to have a basic understanding of this disease, why it occurs, and the general progression we can expect. However, before we begin, you need to have a very clear understanding of one thing: *If you have seen one case of Alzheimer's, you've seen exactly one case of Alzheimer's.* Every single case is different, and it's practically impossible to predict how your loved one's case will progress or how long it will last.

Let's begin by getting one nasty, awful fact about this disease out of the way. *Alzheimer's Dementia is a progressive brain disease that does not get better. Unless something else results in their death prior, it is 100 percent fatal.* There are no survivors of this disease to date. I have heard that we would be better served by calling it "brain failure." We understand heart, liver, and kidney failure. It would seem that "brain failure" would aptly describe the outcome of this disease. I hope the first survivor of this disease has already been born. I hope we get it figured out soon. I am so sorry that it has not happened yet, and that is one reason why I feel compelled to write this book in hopes that it may help you.

This is not a medical textbook, and I have no desire to make it such. I will always try to keep my explanations easily understood by everyone who reads this. If you want more scientific information, I will provide links and other books that you can access in the resources section at the end of this book.

Put into plain English, Alzheimer's Dementia results from plaques and tangles that form in the brain. The plaques are composed of a specific protein that builds up in the brain, much like a plaque builds up in the vessels of the heart and leads to heart disease. This particular type of plaque is a protein-based plaque called amyloid protein. And why this build up occurs in some people and not others (or why it occurs and doesn't develop into AD) is not yet fully understood. Many believe the key to preventing Alzheimer's lies in decoding the mystery of why people develop this protein and how it develops, then use pharmaceuticals to stop it. We've made some progress, but we aren't there yet.

The second component found in the brain of Alzheimer's patients is neurofibullary tangles. In my opinion, these tangles are best described as road blocks in the brain. They prohibit the neurons from firing and making the needed connections to perform everything from making a grocery list to combing our hair.

Both of these taken together cause the death of cells in the brain. Literally, the brain begins to shrink and become visibly smaller on imaging studies. It is this progressive change in the structure and function of the brain that causes the changes we see in those afflicted by Alzheimer's. And the reason no two cases of Alzheimer's are the same is because the changes reflect the exact areas of the brain that the plaques and tangles form (and the resulting cellular death). No two patients have the same exact plaques and tangles in the exact same areas of the brain.

Dementia is a broad category of diseases that affect the brain. Alzheimer's is the most common of those diseases. However, there are more than ninety different forms of dementia, the vast majority of which are quite uncommon. Some of the more common ones outside of Alzheimer's include Parkinson's Dementia, Frontotemporal Lobe Dementia, Lewy-Body Dementia, Huntington's Disease, Krutzfeld-Jakob Disease, Vascular Dementia, and Alchoholic Dementia. There are even times when an individual can have more than one type of dementia occurring simultaneously. For instance, a vascular dementia and Alzheimer's Dementia could occur simultaneously if a person has a restricted blood flow to the brain due to issues with the vasculature of the body and also develops the plaques and tangles associated with Alzheimer's.

Know that many of the differing forms of dementia have some of the same symptoms. So even if your loved one doesn't have Alzheimer's, you can still gain helpful knowledge and insight into their condition and how to help them by reading this book because it is all about meeting them where they are today, working around their own particular set of symptoms, and planning for tomorrow. Also, for ease of reading (and writing), we will just refer to Alzheimer's Dementia as AD from now on. Because AD is the most common form of dementia, this book will largely revolve around the somewhat typical path that the AD patient, and those they love, travel with this disease.

Let's begin by talking about what AD is *not* and how we can distinguish the difference.

Warning signs of AD can often come disguised as the normal cognitive decline (NCD) that most people experience, beginning in about the seventh decade of life. NCD is just that: normal. It does not mean your loved one is developing AD. However, it is important to know the signs of NCD and of AD so that you can distinguish between the two and intervene when and if necessary. Signs of normal cognitive decline include

- Increased processing time, i.e., can get to right answer, it just takes longer.
- Multitasking becomes more difficult, i.e., driving, preparing holiday meals.
- Learning some types of new information can be more difficult, i.e., computers, smart phones.
- Common, everyday tasks take longer.

In short, NCD is normal and is not something to be alarmed by.

Delirium is another example of symptoms that can look like dementia, but it is not. Delirium is reversible and is caused by an infection, illness, chemical deficiency in the body, and more. If you notice a dramatic change in your loved one that mimics dementia or a very sudden worsening of their dementia, consult your primary care physician right away or take them to the emergency department or urgent care. Causes of delirium include

- Urinary tract infection/kidney infection *(This is the number one most common reason. Seek medical help as soon as possible, as it can permanently damage kidneys or turn into sepsis, a very serious medical condition.)*

- Dehydration
- Sleep deprivation
- Medications or combinations of meds
- Encephalitis
- Lyme Disease
- Stroke and other medical emergencies

But chances are, if you really thought your loved one had NCD or delirium, you wouldn't be reading this book. So let's get to it.

2

Signs, Symptoms, and Stages of Alzheimer's Dementia

———————

ACCORDING TO DR. REISBURG of NYU, these are the seven stages of Alzheimer's. There are other staging systems that use three or five stages, but I prefer these seven. Keep in mind that people can exhibit symptoms from more than one stage simultaneously.

Stage 1: No Impairment

The brain is beginning to change, but there is no outward evidence. No one knows the person is developing AD, and there are no medical tests that could detect it at this point.

Stage 2: Very Mild Decline

Memory tests are normal and loved ones don't notice anything yet, but the individual may start to notice that they are having trouble remembering and may find it frustrating. They may even comment about how their memory is declining. I remember a specific Easter Sunday when my mom expressed frustration over not being able to remember things anymore. We didn't notice a thing and reassured her that she had just been too busy getting ready for all of us to come over. When we look back, we now recognize that she was in the second stage of her disease.

Stage 3: Mild Decline
This is the first stage at which testing begins to show a decline. It is now noticeable to family and friends, as well as the patient. Some of the noticeable signs include

- Forgetting a word.
- Difficulty remembering new names or places.
- Difficulty following a recipe.
- Difficulty planning and organizing, such as grocery lists or a holiday function.

Stage 4: Moderate Decline
At this point, the disease is quite apparent and affects everyday living.

- Simple math may become difficult, and so they are unable to accurately manage their finances.
- They may forget details about the distant past or "create" new ones. Family members can mistake this for lying and may be shocked that their loved one is now

lying to them, when they would never have done this previously. They are not lying; it's the disease.
- They may forget to eat and drink adequately.
- Sundowning may be very prevalent during this stage of the disease, and we will address that more in a subsequent section.

Stage 5: Moderately Severe Decline

Here patients start to need help with the everyday tasks of life. Symptoms include

- Difficulty dressing and remembering to bathe themselves.
- Not knowing their address or phone number.
- Significant confusion is often present.

They usually still know their family members and some detail about their childhood and youth. They may have periods during the day where they seem "good" and other times when they are very confused and may become agitated (sundowning). Constant supervision is necessary.

Stage 6: Severe Decline

Patients with the sixth stage of Alzheimer's Disease need constant supervision and frequently require professional care. Symptoms include

- Confusion or unawareness of environment and surroundings.
- Major personality changes.
- Loss of bowel and bladder control.

Stages 7: Very Severe Decline

Stage seven signals impending death. Patients lose physical ability and ability to communicate. They need total care for everything. In this stage, patients often lose their ability or desire to eat and may no longer be able to chew or swallow. Many families worry they are starving or causing their own demise by refusing to eat. I truly believe that the disease no longer allows hunger or thirst cues to be interpreted by the brain. In fact, forcing food into their mouth at this stage can cause choking because the coordination of the muscles needed to chew and swallow is no longer present.

Well, that was depressing. I hate that this book has to deliver things to you that, frankly, you don't want to think about. I truly wish I could spare you. Even after a diagnosis, many family members prefer to stick their heads in the proverbial sand and pretend it is not happening. I get that. I'm pretty sure I was a "sand dweller" at times. In fact, I know I was. It's overwhelming to take in, and occasionally we have to go into self-preservation mode. For most of us, this isn't the only thing we have going on in our lives. We become scared and overwhelmed, and honestly, it is easier not to deal with it some days. Give yourself grace on this issue. But, my friend, I'm going to say this as gently as I can: You cannot stay there with your head in the sand. Failure to act will, I guarantee, result in consequences you did not intend and do not want for your loved one or yourself. That doesn't mean you have to do it alone. There is help, and we will address that later on, too. But you have to push through, and you have to do these things, both for yourself and your loved one.

3

Getting a Diagnosis

———————

PERHAPS YOU ARE reading this book because you believe someone you love may have Alzheimer's or another form of dementia and you don't even know where to start. Others of you have already been hit with a diagnosis. If you have already received a diagnosis, you can likely skip this next section.

To begin, you need to get your loved one to see a physician. For some, this is an easy thing to do because they are going to the physician routinely already. Some never go to a doctor, and it can take a little bit of doing to get them there. But try whatever it takes to get it done, even if they aren't happy about it. It's that important. Remember, there could be other serious issues going on, and once taken care of, the problems could reverse. Please take a moment to contact the physician's office prior to the visit regarding your concerns and please accompany them to the appointment.

Some PCPs (primary care physicians) are quite comfortable with dementia and may even prescribe medications for it. However, if it were me or my loved one, I would ask for a referral to a neurologist or other clinic that specializes in the recognition, testing, and management of Alzheimer's and other forms of dementia. Often, after the testing and diagnosis is complete, they will work with your PCP. They can also make recommendations for care and invoke power of attorney, if necessary.

AD is usually a diagnosis of *exclusion*. That means that we are going to have to rule out all the other possible causes first. For instance, blood work will need to be done, along with an MRI and any other routine medicals tests that are not current. For instance, this could include mammogram and pelvic exam with pap smear for women. Men may need a prostate exam. Everyone will have extensive time into performing cognitive tests and answering many questions and filling out paperwork. You may wonder, why is this all necessary for a memory problem? Well, what if you have brain cancer that is causing the change in cognitive status? Or what if it were breast or another form of cancer that has spread to the brain? It could even be a severe vitamin deficiency. Hence, why it is a diagnosis of exclusion. Everything else simply has to be eliminated because there is no blood test that can done for AD, and in the early states, changes on brain MRI will be difficult to identify.

If all of your medical information is current and your physician feels comfortable that there is not another cause for the decline in memory, they may send you to a specialized doctor known as a neuropsychologist. A neuropsychologist is not a medical doctor but a PhD who specializes in the function of the brain and neurological system. Their services are invaluable for many families who need a diagnosis and information to best help their loved one.

After a day of answering questions, filling out forms, and going through all the other medical tests described above, you will likely be sent home knowing nothing more than when you arrived. You will be scheduled to return at a later date to review all the cognitive testing and results of any medical testing. If you or your loved one has AD or another form of dementia, a doctor or even a team with nurses and others will have the unfortunate task of telling you and your family member(s) that you or your loved one has AD. As gentle as they will try to be, this will be some of the hardest news you've ever had to hear. As I said earlier, for my dad, it was absolutely catastrophic, and he can, almost nine years later, recall everything about that moment and how it felt.

Most likely, they will start your loved one on medication, provide informational pamphlets, and encourage you to get involved in various support groups. You may even receive information about clinical trials that may be occurring at the time. Chances are they will encourage activities that will stimulate the brain—writing, puzzles, and word games—to try and keep the mind as sharp as possible for as long as possible. Exercise may also be encouraged, as it should. They may or may not have you return for follow-up. It is possible that they may send their recommendations to your PCP and all further follow-up is handled there. If you were evaluated by a neuropsychologist, please know that they are not a prescribing physician and they would leave any medications to your PCP.

4

Now What?

MANY PEOPLE LEAVE this situation feeling absolutely overwhelmed and not sure where to turn for help or guidance. And at times, if their loved on is doing "okay" that day, it is quite easy to slip into denial mode. Beware that this is not an uncommon reaction, and you need to guard against it.

First, I would recommend that you assemble your "village." Your children, close friends, and extended family need to be made aware of the diagnosis, and you, the family, need support! Depending on where your loved one is in their journey, you need to spend time talking with them about what they understand is happening to them. Some people are keenly aware and understand their diagnosis. Others, especially if significant time has passed between the first symptoms and diagnosis, are never able to fully grasp what is happening.

Beware that at times, the patient is absolutely certain that there is nothing wrong with *them*. However, on some level, they know they are not performing as they once did. This can cause them to project their frustration onto you, the very person they need the most. They may be suspicious, paranoid, and even accuse you of conspiring with the physicians to "do away with them." Spouses or partners may even be accused of having affairs. If this is the case, you still need to assemble your "village." It's just not going to be able to be with the AD patient in the room. But you need to do it, regardless.

Once you have your people assembled, you need to be brutally honest about the diagnosis and what led to it, if they are not already aware. They need to understand that this is going to be a journey of potentially many years. There are going to be twists, turns, times when you are going to do pretty well and other times when you feel you cannot go on another day. If they ask what they can do, you probably are not going to know what to tell them on that day. So encourage them to check in with you periodically and perhaps even prearrange monthly update meetings or correspondence via email so that everyone can remain aware of what is happening. Also, encourage them to read this book or other books listed in the resource section. As this journey unfolds, you will need increasing amounts of help and emotional support. I want to encourage you to ask for what you need. It truly will be what is best for both you and your loved one.

The stage of life you are in (retired versus still working) and the stage of the disease your loved one is currently experiencing will dramatically affect what comes next. In some cases, this is when the person with AD is "forced" to retire. If you are still working, you may be wondering how long you will be able to continue to leave your partner at home alone (more on that later). If you are both retired, you may be able to continue with many of your usual activities but perhaps at a slower pace. You may notice that you are starting to do more and more around the house. However, encourage the person with AD to still do things that they are capable of doing. For instance, you may now need to prepare lunch, but perhaps they can set the table. Always set them up for success. If they are given tasks that they can no longer complete, it will frustrate them and make them feel inadequate.

If your loved one lives alone, this situation can be even more precarious to navigate. If this is the case and you are not certain if, or for how long, they can remain at home, you need to start discussions with a qualified professional right away. Contact a senior living expert who is also a Certified Senior Advisor. Beware, not all senior living advisors have equal backgrounds or objectives. Carefully choose one you can trust. Ask for references and check their reviews online.

5

Estate Planning, Power of Attorney, and Other Important Matters

———————

FOR ANYONE AND EVERYONE reading this, whether you know someone with dementia, have dementia yourself, or know absolutely no one with dementia, these things need to be discussed, and more importantly, need to be taken care of by each and every one of us. The following things protect us and those we love, and when we are no longer on this Earth, they make things less stressful for those we leave behind.

I cannot tell you how many times we meet with families who have loved ones nearing the end of their time on Earth for a host of reasons only to learn that there are no POAs (Power of Attorney) selected or documents drawn up, a last will and testament does not exist, and no estate planning has been done. I don't pretend to understand why people do not take care of this. I'm not sure if they just assume they will do it "someday," if it's denial of one's own mortality, or if they truly do not understand the importance of it. But whatever the case, there are big consequences for not getting it done.

Power of Attorney—A POA is designated for times when you are unable to make decisions for yourself. A health-care POA makes medical decisions for you when you are no longer able to due to injury, illness, or cognitive status. The same for a financial POA. If you don't have one appointed, one will be appointed for you if it is deemed that you are no longer able to make that decision yourself, so it is best if these documents are in place before they are ever needed.

Many people will appoint a POA for health care and/or finances, and the person appointed often has the erroneous impression that they are able to make decisions for their "person" just based on that designation. That is a myth. Only after the POA has been invoked can the individual act on their behalf. This can be done voluntarily or involuntarily. For instance, some elders decide they no longer wish to have control over their money. They are afraid of being taken advantage of or falling victim to a scam. They can assign their financial POA to a trusted person with the ability to take over the primary responsibility for their finances.

Conversely, when it is found that someone is no longer competent to make decisions, then the POA can be invoked by a physician or other qualified professional. Ironically, if no POA has been appointed prior, often the individual can, in some instances, still appoint a POA even if they have been found to be incompetent. Perhaps they lack the executive function to be able to make financial or health-care decisions for themselves, but if they can demonstrate that they know what a POA is and who they would want to do that for them, one can still be chosen. However, it is still better to be prepared and have these documents executed in advance.

If a physician determines that the individual is no longer competent, this is what happens next:

- If a POA has been appointed, invoke it.
- If not, can they choose?
- If so, assign POA and invoke.
- If not, then a guardianship must be established that has to go through court. (There are emergency guardianships that can usually be established within a few days.)

I hope this helps you to see how important it is to have documents drawn up ahead of time in order to ensure that this will not turn into a large issue for you and your loved ones. If it has been more than five years since your documents were prepared, it is wise to have them reviewed by an attorney, as laws and requirements do change from time to time.

Last Will and Testament—Largely known as a "will." This document serves to control the "who gets what" after your death. This document is only used after the person dies, and it helps ensure that there will not be family disagreements over the outcome. A will is considered binding in a court of law.

Living Will—A living will is different than a Last Will and Testament because it is carried out while the person remains alive. The purpose of a living will is to record the what, when, and how regarding your wish to receive medical treatment or life-sustaining measures. In the event you are unable to communicate those wishes yourself, it allows your family the peace of knowing they did what you would have wanted. It also serves to protect you from unwanted medical interventions or to ensure that you receive medical interventions if you so desire.

Estate Planning—I am not an attorney, nor do I play one on television. Depending on your situation, estate planning can be a complicated matter, and you do need an attorney. I would recommend asking trusted friends, a financial advisor, or a CPA who they would recommend. You can also Google *estate planning attorney* or *elder law attorney*. It will cost you a little bit of money in the short term, but it could save not only money but a great deal of stress in the long term.

6

Restructuring Everyday Life

DURING THE NIGHT after September 11, 2001, I remember holding my then-three-month-old infant, knowing that nothing would ever be the same again. It was my generation's Pearl Harbor. There would forever be a line drawn between the "before" and the "after." I believe life is a lot like that when a diagnosis of cancer, Alzheimer's, or other progressive disease is delivered. You wonder what in the world life will be like now.

If you've recently received an AD diagnosis, then you might be wondering this right now. But I'm going to let you in on a little secret. You've been restructuring your life for a long time already. It just was happening so slowly that you may not have noticed. You have slowly, over time, begun to do more and more for them. If they live with you, you have begun to take on the tasks they once did. If they do not live with you, you may find yourself bringing them groceries, taking them to eat somewhere, stopping by more often, and calling to check on them.

The number one goal of everyday life from here on out is *safety*. Our job in caring for those with dementia is to do everything we can to keep them safe while at the same time preserving their dignity. What does that look like? Remember how there are no two cases of Alzheimer's that look the same? That, unfortunately, makes this and so many other aspects of caregiving such a challenge. No one can write a book that explains, "if this, then that." Perhaps they can no longer execute a grocery list, but they can participate in the making of one and going to the store with you. Perhaps they can no longer keep the garage organized and mow the lawn, but they can walk outside, pull weeds, and help tend to landscaping.

However, if they are trying to use power tools when you are concerned they are no longer safe to do so, it might be time to rehome the tools. Cooking on the stove or using an oven is the same principle. Many families need to disable the stove at some point in order to keep their loved one safe.

Often, the most challenging portion of everyday life is dealing with the incessant, repeated questions or stories. For some, it's the behavior disturbances that often accompany the disease that becomes the most challenging aspect. We will discuss this more in a subsequent section as well.

For the most part, I encourage you to continue everyday life as normally as possible. And this includes the person with dementia as well. If you are still working, continue as long as you are able to or want to. If your loved one needs help or supervision at home, there are people who can come into the home to help. There are also day-stay services available in the community and within memory care facilities.

If your person was accustomed to going to lunch with a group once a month or once a week, then they should continue as long as they can. You are going to need to have a discussion with others about your person and their condition. There is no need to be embarrassed. Chances are they have also known for some time. Give them the opportunity to help you in this way.

One of the most essential aspects of restructuring everyday life is to understand how to communicate effectively with your person. The person with AD is experiencing the death of their brain. With this comes changes in their ability to reason, understand, and remember. Please do not expect them to look at life the same way you do. At times, people will say, "If I could just make her/him understand" or "If I could just get her/him to cooperate." Please hear me on this: That part of their brain is dying or already dead. They would if they could, but they cannot, so please stop expecting them to. It robs them of their dignity and only makes you frustrated. They cannot change, so we must.

We have to dive into their reality. I hate it, but they are not coming back to ours.

But how? I'm so glad you asked. The answer is, "I don't know." It's honestly going to depend on your person. You are going to likely have to try hundreds of different things in order to find what works. Occasionally, you'll get lucky, and with time, you'll start to get better at it. The goal is to preserve their dignity while keeping everyone's frustration to a minimum. Here are some general rules:

1. You have to go into their reality; they cannot join you in yours.
2. You will seldom, if ever, win an argument. They may give up, but they will feel "less than," and what will you have gained? Chances are the only thing you will have gained is to rob them of their dignity. So please, do not argue with your person.
3. They are not trying to be difficult.
4. They are not lying to you. This is their perception of truth now.

So what do we do instead?

1. Acknowledge their point of view and make them feel valued.
2. Redirect to a new task or activity.

3. If they are frustrated, tell them we'll get back to it later and then do something else.
4. Make sure they aren't hungry, ill, tired, or have to use the bathroom.
5. Many people find ice cream or cookies can cure most anything.

It's overwhelming, daunting, and scary. You have to take it one day a time. Often, you will be making it up as you go along. I must warn you, however, that as you get a routine established, with additional time, your person will decline in their ability yet again, and you will have to readjust to yet another new normal. This cycle will continue to play out over and over through the course of the disease.

7

Support for the Caregiver

————————

IF YOU ARE the primary caregiver, then please pass this book along to your support system. I believe it is important for them to have all of this information, and maybe this portion more than any other. The cost of caregiving is high—emotionally, financially, and physically. This is true for any caregiver, but even more so for the caregiver of a dementia patient.

The statistics are staggering. A 2003 study of caregivers by a research team at Ohio State University has proven the oft-repeated adage "stress can kill you" is true. The focus of the investigation was the effect the stress of caregiving had on caregivers. The team, led by Dr. Janice Kiecolt-Glaser, reported on a six-year study of elderly people caring for spouses with Alzheimer's Disease. The study not only found a significant deterioration in the health of caregivers when compared to a similar group of noncaregivers but also found the caregivers had a 63 percent higher death rate than the control group.

Physical cost: The human body is designed to handle sudden and transient stress relatively well. Our "fight or flight" kicks in, and the situation is handled. However, our body is less adept at handling chronic stress. Caregiving, particularly for a dementia patient, produces some of the highest chronic stress levels of all caregivers and perhaps in all of possible life events. The production of increased cortisol (produced by the adrenal glands) has long-term consequences that include but are not limited to increased blood pressure, higher incidence of heart attacks and strokes, weight gain, headaches, and even cancer and much more.

If you are the primary caregiver, you need to be acutely aware of your own needs. The team of people you have assembled need to hear from you about your needs, but they should also be checking in with you. I completely understand that it is difficult to ask for help. Many of us are raised to believe in helping others but not in asking for (or accepting) help ourselves. This is not a sprint. It is a daily marathon, and without help and support, you may not always be able to care for your person for as long as you would like. I'm not joking around about this or being dramatic. It's the plain truth, whether or not you wish to hear it.

Emotional cost: Spouses, partners, adult children, and other family members often put their entire lives on hold in order to become a caregiver for someone with dementia. Some resign from their careers, others give up meaningful activities that provide immense joy and pleasure. Still others sacrifice caring for other family members (children and grandchildren) in order to care for the person with dementia. While this can certainly lead to a feeling of resentment at times, the far greater danger could be the isolation that the caregiver now experiences, having given up so many of the activities they once enjoyed. They slowly become more enveloped into full-time caregiving and spend decreasing amounts of time interacting with anyone other than the patient.

Financial cost: The financial burden of caregiving extends well beyond someone just having to resign from a position. Others cut back on their hours or decline a promotion because they are caregiving. Contributions to retirement are reduced and extra expenses are incurred for medical equipment and supplies or for home modifications and safety measures. Eventually, in-home caregivers are needed, and if the patient is unable to pay, often this falls to other family members as well. Health from the chronic stress of caregiving can decline, thereby increasing the out-of-pocket medical expenses of the caregiver as well.

Please do not ask the person with dementia to understand their dementia. The cruel irony of the disease is it often does not allow the one suffering from it to know they have it.

8

Practical Tips through the Stages

Stage 1—As we discussed earlier, things are happening inside the brain, but the patient is not aware and no one else is aware either. These changes can happen over the course of many years.

Stage 2—At this stage, the patient may begin to become frustrated that they are becoming forgetful. This is difficult, because we all have times that we feel forgetful. Perhaps we are tired or have a virus and we aren't our best. But know that for your person, this is a different feeling for them than the "normal" forgetfulness, and it could potentially show up in frustration that is above and beyond what would be a normal response from them.

But the problem with suggesting any practical tips at this stage is that it will be a rare event when you will be reading this and your person is actually in this stage.

According to John's Hopkins, the average time from onset of symptoms to diagnosis is 2.8 years. That alone would lead me to believe this stage, stage two, may take up a significant portion of those 2.8 years. Based on my knowledge and experience of this disease, this is when you need to be seeking out a diagnosis to clearly identify what is going on. If it isn't Alzheimer's or another form of dementia, early diagnosis and treatment could make all the difference. If it is, then you have the opportunity to make plans for the future, which is an opportunity denied to many who are diagnosed later.

Stage 3—Remember that at this stage, not only does your person know that something is wrong, but it is quite evident at times to others as well. But at other times, you will think they are just fine; and honestly, they will have moments where that is indeed the case. Perhaps repetition is the theme of this stage. Same questions and same stories over and over. You will feel like you've answered the same question countless times in a day, sometimes in the same hour. This may continue throughout the rest of the disease process. But repetition is also a blessing at this stage. Tasks that have been repeated for years, or even over the course of a lifetime, are engrained in the memory that is not as quickly affected. These things can then continue further into the disease.

They will search for words at times. Be patient. Don't be fast to interrupt or correct. Let them see if they can get there. Provide cues when necessary, but know it may not always be appreciated. If they start to become frustrated, try changing the subject or begin a new activity. *Please don't ask them if they can remember this, that, or the other thing.* And please don't assume that just because they remember something one day that they will be able to remember the same thing the next day or the next hour.

You may have a discussion, and they verbally acknowledge and understand what you are saying in that moment. Please don't admonish them if ten minutes later they have no recollection. Remember how I said earlier that Alzheimer's and dementia patients often feel "less than"? How we respond to them in this stage will feed into that for the good or the bad.

There are many things I find ironic about this disease, but perhaps one of the most profound is your person's ability to remember emotions. If something happens that makes them feel scared, hurt, or ashamed, they may indeed hang onto that feeling for a significant period of time. If they get too cold in the bath, they may no longer want to take one. Memories from decades earlier that provoked a strong emotion may also stay with them longer. Some families hear horrific tales from their youth and wonder if there is truth to the story or if it is fiction. I wish I could tell you, but I truly don't know. Perhaps some of both?

Stage 4—Life is beginning to get even more difficult for your person in this stage. They are starting to have fewer and fewer times of lucidity. Hallucinations, delusions, and paranoia may occur in the stage. (Or earlier or later. Remember, no two people experience this disease the same way.) Very scary and traumatic things can happen in this stage. One morning, your spouse of thirty, forty, or even sixty years may wake up and not recognize you. They may ask where their spouse or partner is, and you are standing right in front of them. They may be terrified of you. They may see other people in the house who are not there. This can cause them great distress, thinking that they may need to do something for the "guests" in their home. They may perceive that someone is trying to hurt them.

Our goal as someone who loves them is to help them stay calm and experience peace and joy. How can we take what they perceive to be a scary or stressful situation and bring them joy? Have you ever heard the expression, "throw spaghetti at the wall and see what sticks"? Well, I personally believe that phrase was coined for this disease. You have to try and try until you get it. My mom experienced the frequent hallucination that there were small and even disabled children in her home that she needed to care for. She was often distraught that their parents were not coming to pick them up. I remember my sister took her in another room to distract her, and then when they came out, told her that their parents had come to get them. Mom was so relieved. That piece of spaghetti stuck. We used variations on that approach regularly.

She also accused someone of coming to take her clothes (the "laundry lady") while she was gone. (She was actually "hiding" them herself.) This caused her great distress. So one day, another sister told her to write a note and put it on her clothes that she did not wish for her to "take" them. So she did! Sure enough, when Mom and Dad returned home, the clothes were laying on the bed with the note. Mom was pleased. Stress averted for that moment. Communicate with other members of the care team and family what is working to bring your person peace. This will help everyone, most importantly your person. There are books that are great resources to help you figure some of these things out. They are listed in the resource section of this book.

In this stage you need to begin watching out for every aspect of their lives. They may even forget to eat and drink during this stage. Sometimes your person may seem worse if they are hungry or tired. Alcoholics Anonymous uses the acronym HALT: Hungry, Angry, Lonely, Tired. So true. When your person is struggling, ask yourself if they could be any of those things. (Please also include needing to use the bathroom for AD patients.) When you, the caregiver, are having a difficult time, ask if they could be true for you. Call a time-out. Maybe you both need a nap. Other activities that could help might be a snack, a walk, a movie you both enjoy, or a trip out of the house to visit some friends. (Remember your team? Call one of them if you need to!)

Your patience is going to be tried. They may be argumentative or even mean. They will likely accuse you of things you have never done. (Affairs, trying to harm them, and more.) They may try to walk out the door or even become physically aggressive. They may be fine all day and then suddenly around four p.m. become agitated, restless, and impulsive. This is known as "sundowning," and we'll address that more just a little later.

You have to start leaning on your team. Caregiver burnout is a very real thing because this, my friend, is exhausting. You may feel you are on an island and may be starting to question your own mental capacity, hence the title of this book. You are not alone. Reach out for help. Go to the resource section and get a hold of someone.

It's difficult to even type this, let alone live through it. I wish I didn't have to. But please hear me when I say this is why you absolutely must have a team in place. You cannot do this alone.

If your person resides alone, they simply cannot do so at this point. They need 24/7 supervision. They are a danger to themselves and to others. They may eat rotten food or not eat at all. They may leave the stove on, burn food they are trying to prepare, forget to pay the gas bill, thus leaving them without heat or even water and phone. In reality, they shouldn't have been residing alone before now, but at this stage, it is imperative. We'll cover more about memory care later on, but I did feel it important to mention at this point.

"The person with dementia is not giving you a hard time. The person with dementia is having a hard time."
—*Unknown*

Stage 5—Significant sundowning is often present in this stage of the disease (and sooner), so the tactics you are able to employ from six a.m. to four p.m. may be completely different than from four p.m. until they are asleep. Speaking of sleep... Sleep disturbances are quite prevalent with AD. Some patients sleep a lot; others seem to hardly ever sleep. Still others will completely confuse their nights and days. Keeping to a routine and having plenty for your person to occupy themselves with is important. While they can no longer accomplish the tasks they once did, they still have need to stimulate all five senses.

Music is a wonderful tool in all of the stages, but in this stage, it can literally bring them peace and joy. Sometimes even memories will come back of times long ago. Singing together, looking at old photographs, simple crafts and flowers are a few other things that come to mind. In my humble opinion, cookies or ice cream can cure almost anything. When things get rough, try, "I think some ice cream sounds wonderful right now. I would love for you to join me," and see if that helps. It may, in fact, help both of you.

The person you once knew is now rendered almost childlike in their dependence upon you. The few chores they were able to do before may now be lost. They will rely upon you for bathing, dressing, preparing food, and all the other essentials of daily life. However, when you hand them the toothbrush, they may still be able to remember what to do. If you hand them a comb or a shirt, likewise. But without the cues coming from you, they will not be able to recall the tasks that need to be done.

They may flat-out refuse as well, despite the cues from you. (Ah, yes ... if only all Alzheimer's patients were sweet and compliant. In my experience that may be more the exception than the rule.) When they refuse, you must then decide if this is a hill you want to die on, so to speak. Do they insist on wearing the same thing? Is it possible to accommodate if this makes them happy? Could you possibly wash at night or buy more than one? On the other hand, if they refuse to bathe, this can get a little more tricky. Sometimes keeping the room warmer can help. Other times you may need to hire a caregiver to come in and bathe your person while you step out to run errands, enjoy a walk, or have a cup of coffee with a friend. Does that make sense? Of course, if it is a matter of safety, then yes, you need to keep them safe at all costs, while at the same time keeping yourself safe and sane.

Stage 6—In stage six, your person may not be talking much anymore. Even the simplest of tasks are no longer able to be completed. Cues for brushing hair or teeth may no longer work. Using utensils to eat may not work and attempting to eat nonedibles may come into play. (This may happen sooner as well.) They may be less agitated at times or more agitated. Again, it just depends. But as they journey through stage six, they will need assistance for absolutely everything. Keeping adequate hydration is essential in stage six, and you will need to encourage your person to drink by offering their favorite things or even popsicles and other foods high in water content.

Their motor skills are going to start waning at this point because the disease is progressed enough that the signals from the brain to the extremities are hindered. And the less they use them, the weaker they become, and the more susceptible your person will become to falling and other accidents. Safety from falling, choking, and walking out the door into traffic is paramount.

Tips at this point? Get help. Plain and simple. It's not pretty. Use music; sit and hold their hand. Give them something to hold in their hands. Some people like to hold a stuffed animal or even a baby doll for comfort (even before this stage). If they believe their parents are alive or that you are their parent, just go with it. Whatever makes them happy and at peace. Provide a lot of verbal reassurance.

I would be remiss if I didn't devote at least one paragraph to the subject of urinary tract infections (UTIs). This may sound odd to you, but as Alzheimer's progresses, UTIs become quite common and can have surprising consequences. At any time during this disease, when someone develops a UTI, they can have a serious and dramatic change in cognitive status. Same goes for other infections and viruses, but when you see this type of sudden change, always be thinking UTI. Easy to rule out and treat, but not so easy to spot outside of the cognitive changes. As people age, UTIs become less and less symptomatic. It's almost like it is an insidious little monster waiting to show up. One morning, your person who is in stage five or six may not be able to be aroused to wake. Or they suddenly may not be able to walk or cannot say any coherent words. Be on the lookout for this, and call your doctor right away. They will likely return to their previous status once the infection has cleared.

Stage 7—Your person will still be with you in body at this stage, but they are no longer going to be able to interact with you. These are the final weeks and days. You may certainly offer food and drink, but they may not always be interested. They may now lack the ability to coordinate the chewing and swallowing of food, so be very cautious in this stage in regard to choking. They are helpless and often unable to walk or even talk.

Do what you think would offer them comfort and what comforts you. Perhaps reading from their favorite book, playing music or singing songs, sitting with them, pushing them in their wheelchair outside on a nice day, and just enjoying. Not always but often they are at peace in this stage, peace which may have eluded them in earlier stages.

Bring family and friends around to visit with you and to share their memories of wonderful times together. Perhaps a favorite blanket or pillow. Let them know you are there and that they are not alone. Their journey is nearly complete. They may no longer remember you, but always assure them that you remember the wonderful person they are.

A word about hospice... This word tends to frighten people because to them it means death. When your person is in the fifth and sixth stages of dementia, it is time to think about something known at palliative care and hospice. As much as I hate it, Alzheimer's is fatal 100 percent of the time. There are no survivors. I want to encourage you to consider how you would want your last days to go. One of the reasons I advocate for early diagnosis is so you can have discussions about things such as this very subject. Sometimes it does not always work out that way, however, and you will need to use your best judgement.

Palliative care and hospice often work in conjunction with each other to bring the highest quality of life for the patient. Notice I did not say the highest quality *death*. This is about life. It does not have to mean impending death when it is started a little earlier. It simply gives another layer of support for you and your loved one. I recommend interviewing two or more hospice providers to learn of their particular philosophy toward the hospice process. Share with them your beliefs and wishes regarding end of life for your person and ask as many questions as you need to feel comfortable. In my personal experience, hospice is not a scary thing but rather a tremendous blessing.

More on this subject a little later.

9

Living Arrangements

———

THERE ARE PROBABLY as many ways to do this as there are people who do it. There is no one right or wrong answer on this. If you choose to care for your loved one for a period of time, deep into the disease, or not at all, you are wonderful! One is not better than the other. Not being the primary caregiver does not make you any less of a person or mean you have less love than the one who cares far, far into the disease. Admitting that caregiving is not for you may actually be the best way for you to care for them. And that is okay. There is no way I can cover every situation here, but allow me to give you some scenarios.

John and Marie are in their late seventies. John and their adult children have noticed changes in Marie for several years, and she has now been diagnosed with Alzheimer's. She was between stages three and four at the time of diagnosis. John cared for her and was able to leave her at home for short periods of time. Eventually, John's children let him know that he should no longer leave her alone. They helped him hire private-duty caregivers to be with her while he enjoys some recreational activities or spending time with friends. Marie is a sweet and compliant patient for John. She is almost always agreeable. John is in good health, and Marie is a small lady. He is able to help her bathe and dress, and he does all the cooking and laundry. This arrangement continues for several years. Marie begins to lose control of bowel and bladder, but John refuses to give up caring for her. One morning, Marie is unable to be awakened. She is taken by ambulance to the ED, where she is diagnosed with a UTI. John takes her home after she responded favorably to fluids and antibiotics. Less than thirty days later, it happens again, at which time John relents, at his children's urging, and Marie is placed into care from the ED. They were not able to get their first choice for Marie, and they had to place in her a town twenty minutes away.

Susan is in her sixties and has no living family that she remains in contact with. Friends have been noticing odd behavior and have tried to help her, but she pushes them away. Her closest friend breaks contact with her, hoping that she will finally reach out for help. Susan goes to people at the church she attends and reaches out for assistance but confesses that she doesn't understand why she can't seem to remember at times. Susan continues to go to work and drives. (She was about to lose her job and had gotten lost on more than one occasion.) One hot summer afternoon, her car stalled, and she walked a significant distance to the church. Once inside the doors, she collapsed. She was hospitalized for dehydration, malnutrition, and confusion. During her hospitalization, she is declared unable to make medical or financial decisions for herself. Her closest friend reenters the picture and agrees to take on the role of POA. Susan is placed into memory care, where there are several other patients her age.

Richard and Doris are sixty-five and fifty-seven, respectively. Richard has Alzheimer's and is retired. Doris still works full time and needs to continue for economic reasons, and she thoroughly enjoys her job. Recently, Richard reached the point in his journey where he is no longer able to be left alone. At first, they brought in private caregivers, but they could not afford to have them in the home forty hours a week. They located a memory support community that offered day-stay services at significantly less cost. (Day stay is often referred to as adult day care. I loathe that term and feel it robs people of their dignity.) Richard spends his days engaged with others and in meaningful activities, gets nutritious food, and sleeps well at night. When the time comes that Richard needs 24/7 memory support, it will be a very easy transition as he will already feel "at home" there.

Connie and Paul have been married for fifteen years. This is a second marriage for both of them, and there are grown children from previous marriages. Paul has had some dementia for several years, but recently it has become much worse. He is isolating himself and does little else other than watch TV. He is verbally hostile to his children and wife. His son finally had to take his keys away after Connie became very scared while riding in the car with him. Paul became outraged, and while his son had taken the keys, he blamed Connie. The family attempted to talk to Paul about the need to possibly relocate with Connie to a senior living community where they could "age in place." (They knew that Paul would eventually need memory care.) He refused to consider this option and became more and more angry. One afternoon, he stormed out of the house after yelling at Connie. Because of the size difference as well as his intense anger, Connie was unable to keep him from leaving. Family and authorities were called. Paul was located several hours later after utilizing both dogs and helicopters. He had walked more than five miles from his home in chilly conditions. He was hospitalized in a senior mental health unit. From there, the family was able to place him into memory care. He was extremely angry with his children and with Connie for several months. However, he is now settled in his environment and thriving with the activities and support he receives. He loves to have his wife and family visit.

Lilian is a ninety-three-year-old widow who had been living alone for many years. Lilian had a history of mental illness, likely undiagnosed bipolar disorder. She had one grown son who lived many hours away by car. He visited as he could, but was somewhat reluctant to do so because of her history of erratic behavior. He was also busy running his own company in another state. Always given to "hoarding tendencies," as Lilian aged and then developed Alzheimer's, the hoarding became significantly worse. Eventually, her son hired private in-home caregivers who immediately assessed that the situation was unsafe. The help of a Certified Senior Advisor was called. Lilian insisted that there was absolutely nothing wrong with her and that everyone was conspiring to "put her away." She continued to insist on driving herself to the store. The son eventually "disabled" the car so that she could not leave with it. She spent her days in a kitchen chair, where she looked out the window while listening to the local AM radio station. There was literally no other place to sit in the home, and the shortest stack that lined the path from door to table to bedroom and bathroom was nearly four feet tall. One tiny space was free to sleep on the bed, otherwise there was no open space in the entire three-bedroom home. With the enticement of a free lunch, Lilian and her son accompanied the senior advisor to several memory care communities. One in particular seems to strike a chord with Lilian. She was smiling and visiting with the other residents and commented often how beautiful it was. The son decided that this would be the most beneficial community for his mother, and arrangements were made for her to move in.

Unfortunately, the cruelty of the disease prohibited Lilian from remembering the positive experience she had at the community, and when it was time to move, she protested and stated that no one was going to remove her from her home. When the senior advisor arrived at the home, Lilian was gently reminded of the need for her to be safe and how much her son worries about her. Lilian complained that no one had let her pack. (She had helped pack the previous day.) The advisor recommended that she get busy packing! Lilian picked out several things to put in a small bag that she wished to take along. Lilian then went willingly to the community, holding her bag of items tightly the whole way. While Lilian would often complain that her son had just "dropped her off and left her there," she thrived in the safe, clean, and socially stimulating environment.

Janice is sixty-six and has been cared for by her loving husband, Tim, since her diagnosis at sixty-one. Tim cared for Janice alone until he could no longer leave her home alone while he went to work. They brought in private-duty nonmedical in-home caregivers to stay with her while he was away. One morning while Tim was helping Janice shower, she started screaming. She didn't recognize him and thought there was a strange man attacking her in the shower. Tim's heart was broken. He also noticed that she was becoming more and more depressed and realized that she needed more interaction and stimulation. He knew it was time for her to move into a memory care community. He and his daughter selected a loving environment with social activities and plenty of space for her to walk and enjoy the outdoors, all while being protected and kept safe.

When my family was taking the journey through this disease, we often heard our dad comment that mom would have to "get much worse" before she would be able to handle living in the memory care community. I believe now that this was our "code" for "we have to wait until she is so bad that she won't know what is happening." While placing a loved one into a memory care community prior to this point in the disease may both sound and feel counterintuitive, it's actually very beneficial at times. There is no one right or wrong way to do this, and it is certainly not a one-size-fits-all formula. Remember that at some level the person with dementia or Alzheimer's recognizes that they are not like everyone else and can feel "less than" when they cannot keep up with conversations and activities like they once may have. As discussed earlier, this can lead to self-isolation, depression, and a lack of self-worth.

In a memory care community, everyone is like them. Every moment of every day is structured to meet the person exactly where they are in their journey, and they are celebrated for being exactly who they are. Many people sense a deep relaxing exhale when they are surrounded by peers who are like themselves. The structure of the routine brings comfort and predictability to their days. Stimulating the five senses during the day and getting exercise, their normal medications, and good nutrition can lead to better sleeping patterns at night, which further improves their overall health and well-being. And if they cannot sleep well at night? Well, someone is always there to assist them, drink a warm cup of tea, or just walk the halls with them. And you, their loved ones? Now you, too, are getting a good night's sleep. When you visit, you are no longer the caregiver but the family member, spouse, or friend once again. As long as they are able, you can even take them for shopping trips, family gatherings, and holidays.

When a person moves while they still are able to interact, carry on meaningful conversations, and participate in activities, they are able to adapt and learn to call the community their new "home." As the disease progresses, they are already settled into the environment and familiar with the staff, and they will generally do well for a longer period of time. Perhaps counterintuitive, but it's been borne out time and time again. The reasons and timing for entering into a memory care community are as numerous as the families affected by this disease. Differing circumstances make it easier or more difficult to care for people in their homes. As you read in the examples, the experience is different for everyone. Lean on your team to help you decide when it may be time to get help into the home and when it's time to move.

As we discussed, individuals with AD are very reluctant and even obstinate about moving. Again, this can get a little bit tricky! There are many tactics we employ to help make this easier on you and the family. My personal favorite is to throw people under the bus—everyone except the family and close friends, that is. The doctors, the senior living advisor, the plumbing, the weather, and the list goes on. In addition, we suggest bringing your person to the memory care community for day-stay services, if possible, before moving in. When we have incorporated this strategy, it has worked exceptionally well. Half days turn into full days, and eventually they stay for night. Granted, we don't always have this luxury. A good memory care community will also help you in every way possible to make this transition easier for your person. This may be your first foray into this experience, but the experts know how to make this work. Lean on them.

The transition into memory care will be harder for you than for the patient. Give it time.

10

Assisted Living and Memory Care

———

MANY FAMILIES ARE worried that their person will be mad at them. Sometimes this is the case. However, if there is a blessing inside this cruel disease, it is their ability to forget, at least in this instance. The vast majority of AD patients will adjust and cease to be mad within a few weeks. They may still ask to go home every time you see them. But when this is explored further, "home" ends up meaning many things and can even be their childhood home or a place they lived decades before. That word, "home," and when they plead with us to take them there can stir up powerful emotions within us and make us feel horrible for having them in memory care. However, remember that our number one job is to keep them safe. Give it some time and ask the staff for help. Someone you can talk to who has experienced this themselves would also be most helpful. Many memory care communities form a "family" of support to help each other, which is a wonderful added benefit.

Sundowning

I've referred to this term several times in the course of the book, and I wanted to devote a little extra time to the subject. If you are not already familiar with the phenomenon, you may think this sounds a little bit like Greek right now, but trust me when I say a high percentage of AD patients experience sundowning.

During the later parts of the day, typically around three p.m. or after, there seems to be a shift in the demeanor and personality of many of those afflicted with AD. It is believed that this is caused by the fading sunlight. Some AD patients can do quite well in the earlier hours of the day but present entirely different in the late afternoon and evening. What makes this particularly challenging is the time of day that your person may end up seeing their physician ... most of those occur in the morning or early afternoon. It is the experience of this practitioner that often our physicians don't see the true spectrum of the disease as it affects families and loved ones because of this simple scheduling issue.

While this phenomenon does not occur in all patients, it is likely more common than not, at least on some level.

Some signs of sundowning that may occur alone or together include

1. Exit seeking. They feel the need to go somewhere and do something at this time of day. Perhaps because this is when they left work to go home, had to go to school to get the children, had to complete chores on the farm, etc. Letting them know that the "kids are home," the "hired hand did the chores already," or that they should "come, sit, and put their feet up after a hard day at the office," is enough to remove the compelling force to try and leave.
2. Confusion and/or agitation increases.
3. They may become sad or tearful.
4. They may pace, fidget, or seek out other people to be around.
5. Speech may become more difficult to understand, incontinence may increase, and they may have more difficulty making their needs known.

Of course, it's great to recognize the symptoms of sundowning, but the real question is how do we handle it? Sundowning leads to increased anxiety in our loved one, and our goal is to minimize that as much as possible, thereby giving them peace and comfort while at the same time reducing our own level of stress and frustration.

Since there is often a compelling urge to move around when sundowning and to be near other people, take advantage of that propensity and use it to your advantage. If your person is able-bodied, go for a walk with them, have them help with dinner (what they are safely able to do successfully), or put on some music and dance! You may have to try several different approaches to find what works for your person. (More spaghetti throwing!) However, as many so often find, and as I've said many times already, ice cream or cookies will solve almost anything.

11

End-of-Life Decisions

———

BECAUSE EACH CASE of AD is different from the next, there is no way to predict how long it will take for the disease to run its inevitable course. The time each person stays in the various stages will differ. The best time to have these discussions is before any one would ever become ill with a terminal disease. Please heed this advice and put your wishes in writing. Consult with an elder law professional to help you through this process. However, if that has not been done, and if your person was/is too far into the disease to express verbally or in writing what their wishes would be for this time in their life, then you will have some decisions to make.

As the disease progresses into the final stages, motor skills will begin to decline. The disease that has caused so much brain tissue to die will begin to affect balance, coordination, and even chewing and swallowing. A wheelchair will become necessary. Eating will slow down or stop altogether. Palliative and hospice care is often initiated. Let's talk about each of those services. Most people are frightened at the mention of either of them, as they often bring with them the notion of imminent death.

Palliative care focuses on comfort and alleviating any symptoms that may be causing distress for the patient. Palliative care shares a similar philosophy with hospice, but palliative care can also exist separately from hospice. Palliative care focuses on advanced planning and symptom management while still receiving active treatment. Palliative care helps to provide clear information about your health-care options, guidance in your choice, and assistance in collaboration with your primary physician. Palliative care typically pursues a path to hospice when the individual and/or their families are ready to stop active treatment. For example, if trying to get medications into your person only results in a "fight," if you will, then maybe it's time to review with their physician. However, if some of their medications help them feel better or experience less distress, then perhaps an alternate route, such as topical or even mixing them in with food, could be explored.

Another example of palliative care would be to explore all of their doctor's appointments. At this stage of the disease, you may want to reconsider if they still need to attend appointments with their ophthalmologist or dentist. Of course, if you or their caregiver perceives that they are in discomfort or pain, you will want to address that, but if not, consider that going out and seeing these providers may very well cause more angst in this stage of the disease.

Hospice is generally deemed appropriate when an individual is determined to have six or fewer months to live. This is not a rule set in stone. People often live many months on hospice. I say this because it is not something to be feared. Hospice does not have to be a "call the family because it's almost over" situation. Hospice opens a door for additional benefits and is covered 100 percent by both Medicare and traditional insurance. Hospice provides all medical equipment, like a specialized bed, wheelchair, and incontinence products, and hospice pays for all medications related to the terminal illness and comfort. Hospice provides nursing, a nursing aide, a social worker, a spiritual counselor, and volunteers who will play music or just sit with your loved one.

Hospice is not a *place*. Hospice is a service that comes to you wherever your loved one is. That can occur in your home, in a memory care community, the hospital, or even a hospice house. Hospice also does not provide round-the-clock caregivers. Depending on your individual needs and plan of care, a hospice provider will come at regular intervals but will be available to you 24 hours a day. Hospice aides will also come at regular intervals to help with bathing and personal hygiene, depending on the patient's needs. If you and your loved one need additional care over that and you are not in a memory care community or another community with round-the-clock care, you will need to hire private-duty caregivers. This is not covered by Medicare or personal health insurance.

Many people associate hospice with the use of powerful narcotics and other medications they believe may hasten the process of dying. Let me be very clear when I say *you are in control* of what medications are used and when they are used. Many medications help ease discomfort and anxiety. Your hospice team will educate you on the medications, their function, and possible side effects. The hospice team will communicate openly and honestly with you. If your loved one is in memory care or a skilled nursing community, you will want this communication to extend to them as well. Have frank and open discussions with the staff there about your wishes and needs. Communication is key.

This is hard stuff, and this will be a very difficult time to negotiate. You are getting ready to say goodbye. I've known people who in these very later stages of AD have begun tube-feedings and other measures to keep their person with them longer. This is a very personal decision, and I do not pretend to have the answers for you or your loved one. When people seek out my counsel in these situations and wonder what they should do, I simply state the following:

The thing you need to ask yourself is, are you prolonging life or are you prolonging death?

I do not have the answer to that question, either, and it is likely different for each person facing these decisions. But when you yourself feel that you have crossed over from prolonging life to prolonging death, then it's time to let go and focus on keeping your loved one comfortable and experiencing the highest quality of life and dignity that you can possibly give them.

Another issue that often comes up in this final stage is that of hunger and dehydration. When they refuse to eat and drink, people understandably worry that their loved one is suffering. While I can't prove it, I honestly don't think my own mother could recognize those signals any longer. Her brain was so ravaged by disease that she no longer felt hunger or thirst. And while it sounds cruel, natural dehydration is actually a very humane and even gentle way to leave us. Please hear my heart that I understand if you cannot do this, for whatever reason. But before we had tube-feedings and IVs, the human body was very adept at taking care of these things.

In these final weeks and days, sit with them. Talk to them. Play music, sing, and read whatever would bring comfort to them and to you.

12

Grieving

I ERRONEOUSLY THOUGHT that since I had already been living the slow, torturous loss of my mother over many, many years, I had done all the grieving I would need to do. I thought that I would be so relieved her suffering was over that this would be a very smooth transition for me. I have never been so wrong.

Yes, this disease requires much grieving before they leave us physically, but for some of us, the final goodbye brings with it a finality for which we are ill prepared. Everyone grieves differently. Some appear not to grieve at all because they internalize it or, for whatever reason, just do not show the outward signs like others do. Others grieve in a more outward manner that is visible to others.

Here are a few things I've learned about grief:

1. Probably the most important thing I've ever learned about grief was shared with me by a dear friend from my youth shortly before my mom passed away. I share this with others at least once a week and sometimes more: "With grief, there are no rules." It is your grief process, which will be as unique as the person you loved. I am giving you permission to feel whatever you feel whenever you feel it. No judgment.

2. Grief is the badge of honor we are privileged to wear as the result of great love. Where there is no love, there are no tears. Of course, you can grieve without tears. Remember, is it your journey. No judgment.

3. Some people are what I call "delayed grievers." I am one of them. I don't grieve at the time I'm expected to grieve. But a few weeks later, it will hit in full force and catch me by surprise.

4. "Brain in the Blender" syndrome is real. It's what I call the fog that makes our brains "wonky" with great loss. Simple tasks leave us helpless, we can't make decisions, and we feel like we cannot remember our own names. Be patient with yourself. This will get better with time.

5. Distraction can be a blessing. While it doesn't negate our grief, I would be lying if I didn't say that I needed a break from grieving at times! Maybe it's a good comedy, a night out, or a short trip out of town. And it's

okay if you catch yourself having a good time and even "forgetting" for a bit.

6. There will be days. Days that you cannot function. I give you permission to not "function" for a time. However, be cautious with this. If you are going down to a place that you feel is not healthy for you, please seek help. Friends, this is where we need to care for one another. Are you concerned for someone who is grieving? Do not ignore this! Reach out to them, love them, and help them find the assistance they need.

7. With time, the sharpness of grief will begin to soften. When? I have no idea. It's your journey and there are no rules, remember? In my experience, it never goes away, but I felt as if I began to adapt to the new path I was on. Not without grief but with grief. And I discovered that life can still be increasingly beautiful, not just with grief but perhaps because of it.

8. For some, the real grieving process does not even begin for weeks following the loss. Often, we are thrown into a flurry of activity. There may be a service to plan, family that comes from out of town, thank-yous to write, and casserole dishes to return. As the weeks and months passed, grief may start to become more intense.

"There is a sacredness in tears. They are not a mark of weakness, but of power. They speak more eloquently than ten thousand tongues. They are the messengers of overwhelming grief, of deep contrition and of unspeakable love."

—Unknown

13

Where We Are Going

————————

WE'VE MADE SOME progress, but have a long way to go. We have a few medications that may slow down the progression of the disease for some people. We've come up with new formulations to make dosing easier. But to date, we lack the "magic bullet" that can stop or even reverse the disease.

Genes have been identified that may predispose some individuals to the development of AD, both early and late onset. This may come as useful information to some and completely terrify others. Whether or not you want to know your predisposition to this disease is a discussion to be held with your family and your health-care provider. I myself am hesitant. But my health-care provider pointed out that the information could be useful retrospectively for researchers to learn more about why some people develop the disease and others don't. Something to consider. I still haven't made up my mind.

We have gotten a lot better at caring for those suffering with the disease. To date, it is my opinion that the most progress has been made in this area. We no longer tie individuals to their wheelchair and leave them in large geriatric wards with little to do other than wait for the next meal to be served. We've learned the art of bringing dignity to the world of those afflicted with dementia. We now understand that stimulating all five senses, helping them continue to give back to others, and building their self-esteem by emphasizing what they have rather than what they have lost is a much better way to go. Memory care communities are beautiful places with stimulating activities, gardens, and walking paths where dignity, safety, and compassionate care are found.

Resources, organizations, and support groups exist for family members faced with this diagnosis. It's no longer taboo to talk about dementia or admit that our loved one has been diagnosed. Even fifty years ago, this was not something spoken of outside of immediate family (if even that). The person suffering from the disease was merely "old," "senile," or had "hardening of the arteries." While people understand and recognize AD as a disease affecting memory, we still have much education to do with families and the public at large on how the disease actually works. Unless they have dealt with it personally, most people have many misconceptions about the disease.

My hope is that this book will serve to help you in your own personal education about this disease. If you now feel better able to serve or care for someone with this disease as a result of reading this book, then my mission will have been accomplished. Unfortunately, there is no way to cover every topic or address every scenario within these pages. It is meant to be a starting point. The next section has resources listed that you can use to broaden your understanding even more. I sincerely hope you will take advantage of many of them.

Resources

Books

The 36-Hour Day: A Family Guide to Caring for People Who Have Alzheimer Disease, Related Dementias, and Memory Loss by Nancy L. Mace and Peter V. Rabins

Creating Moments of Joy along the Alzheimer's Journey: A Guide for Families and Caregivers by Jolene Brackey

Dementia Caregiver Guide by Teepa Snow

Learning to Speak Alzheimer's: A Groundbreaking Approach for Everyone Dealing with the Disease by Joanne Koenig Coste and Robert Butler (foreword)

Still Alice by Lisa Genova

Blogs

alzheimersreadingroom.com

alzheimersweekly.com

bakingandbutterflies.wordpress.com

YouTube Channels
Careblazers: Dementia Care Heroes

Teepa Snow's Positive Approach to Care

Podcasts
The Alzheimer's Podcast with Mike Good of Together in This

Dementia Care Partner Talk Show with Teepa Snow

Websites
alz.org

caregiver.org

To Find a Certified Senior Advisor Near You
csa.org

OasisSeniorAdvisors.com

Discussion Questions

With the person diagnosed with AD:

Tell me how you feel your memory is.

Do you think your memory is better or worse than it used to be? (*If they have no comprehension that there is an issue with their memory, do not go any further with them. Pick a different time of day and try again. If the result is the same, it would be my advice to discontinue asking them about it.*)

If they have an understanding of what is happening to them:

What does your worsening memory mean for your/our future?

How do you want to be cared for?

If something happens to me (primary caregiver) or if it no longer works to be at home, what are your wishes then?

Do you have certain cares you would not want your primary caregiver to perform for you? *(Some examples may include toileting, showering, etc.)*

How do you feel about having someone come to the house to care for you when you can no longer stay alone?

Review POA and other legal documents to make sure that they remain comfortable with their choices.

Review end-of-life wishes and funeral arrangements.

As a family or team without the person diagnosed with AD:

Is everyone aware of the diagnosis and what it means?

What are the strengths that everyone brings to the table to help? *(Not everyone is a caregiver. Some are good at planning, others may wish to help with household chores or finances.)*

How often will we meet to discuss how things are going? *(In person or electronically.)*

Is the primary caregiver comfortable being "called out" by other members when they are worried about his or her physical or emotional health?

Are members comfortable with being "called out" if they are slipping into denial or other unhealthy behaviors?

Are members prepared for times when the primary caregiver may need emergency relief? Is the primary caregiver comfortable reaching out when it is needed?

Are there specific parameters that can be identified now that will necessitate a move to memory care? (It may be easier to do this early and then have it agreed to by the primary caregiver. Later, the emotions of the situation may cloud judgment.)

Are all legal documents in place and does everyone understand what their role may (or may not) entail?

How will big decisions be handled? Simple majority? Super majority? Primary caregiver has the final say?

Can you all pledge to put the person with AD and their needs ahead of your own?

About the Author

Beth Friesen is a Registered Nurse, Certified Alzheimer's Disease and Dementia Care Trainer, Certified Dementia Practitioner, and Certified Senior Advisor. She owns and operates Oasis Senior Advisors in Lincoln, Nebraska, where she works with families to assist them in identifying the best senior living options to meet their needs. She spends considerable time educating and counseling families directly affected by the various forms of dementia, as well as other challenges of aging.

Shortly before her mother broke free of Alzheimer's Disease and entered Eternal Life, her mom challenged her to "take good care of your people." By helping individual families, as well as teaching and training others to impact the lives of those living with Alzheimer's Disease and other dementias, Beth hopes to fulfill the promise she made and ultimately fulfill the mission to which she has been called.

Beth and her husband make their home in Lincoln, Nebraska. They have three grown children, a son-in-law, and one silly little dog. In additional to teaching, training, and writing, Beth enjoys fitness, traveling, and sunset watching.

To learn more or to book Beth for your next event, visit her website at www.BethFriesenRN.com or email her at info@BethFriesenRN.com.

CPSIA information can be obtained
at www.ICGtesting.com
Printed in the USA
BVHW041422181119
564177BV00022B/2158/P